Pain in the Back

Effective healing remedies to

Cure chronic back pain

Russell Davis

Table of Contents

Chapter 1

Back Discomfort and a Few Well-Known Triggers

There are many men and women who are struggling with back problems, however that does not suggest that you need to endure it or purchase creams or prescription medications to handle it. You will find that there are plenty of treatments and other helpful options which will assist you in getting your back aches in check, and minimizing your chances of another occurrence even if you are struggling with continuous back troubles. Anybody can experience back discomfort, no matter your age or what part of the planet you live on. Unfortunately, back problems really become more prevalent as we get older, and lots of folks start to notice the aches and discomfort in their backs somewhere near their mid-thirties.

Typical Reasons Why people Experience Back Pain:

If you are the type who does not enjoy a lot of exercise, then you may have a higher probability of experiencing back discomfort than people who are generally in shape. A second element to consider that places you with an increased chance of back soreness is being too heavy, which is the key reason why sustaining a healthy size will enable you to control your back pain if you are currently experiencing it. The reason for this is that an excessive amount of pounds adds tension and pressure to your back, which can certainly trigger long-term discomfort.

Unfortunately, a person can be more susceptible to back problems due to their family genes. Inherited genetics plays a big part as-well, particularly if joint inflammation has a history within the members of your family. There are several forms of joint disease that have an impact on the vertebrae. For those who have an occupation that involves a lot of heavy lifting, twisting, or standing for long periods of time, then it is highly likely that this will also add to your back problems. Poor form when lifting, standing or sitting may furthermore add to flare-ups happening again. Another poor habit that can cause back troubles is smoking cigarettes. The reason for this that smoking cigarettes may prohibit important vitamins and minerals that are needed in order to maintain a healthy spine, not to mention smoking is a gross habit. So do your wallet and your back a favor and do away with the cigs.

Realizing When It's Time to Deal with It:

A person must by no means allow their back troubles to escalate to a serious condition, this is why it is vital to begin with the necessary treatments as early as possible to prevent ongoing problems. Perhaps you may encounter aches and pains that do not improve when you sleep, then that is a sure sign that you should consider finding a solution. If you have a pins and needles sensation in your lower back or down through the back of your legs, then that is a sure sign to start seeking out help.

Again, if you find yourself suffering from stress or tension in your back, then it is definitely time to seek out a solution before the problem worsens. In fact, minimal back problems can also be addressed using healthy techniques. In the event that your back issues are hindering you from doing some of the things that you would like to do, then you need to take care of it immediately. So if you are having trouble resting, can't drive for periods of time without stopping to stretch, or having difficulty making it through your day at work, then your back deserves serious attention and there are natural remedies that we will discuss in this book that will help you!

Chapter 2

Herbal Teas that can assist in Alleviating Back Aches

Sometimes a cozy hot cup of tea is just the relief you need to help ease away any discomfort in your back. By drinking this appropriate blend of tea, you will find that it focuses on your back soreness and provides fast relief. These simple herbal blends are hassle-free beverages that intended to be sipped while hot for maximum effectiveness. Nevertheless, a few folks also enjoy them on ice instead.

#1 Herbal Tea - Pain Reducing Mixture

Combining these ingredients will help to alleviate any soreness in your back rather quickly. Inflammation in your muscles is the primary reason that most people suffer from continuous back aches. Feel free to consume this blend as a day to day routine. If you feel that you need more than one cup, then drink more of this tea as you need it. The combinations of turmeric and ginger have proven to be a very good solution for reducing back pain.

Ingredients:

1. 2 tablespoons of grated ginger

2. 1 teaspoon of turmeric powder

3. 1 cup of water

4. 2 teaspoons of raw honey

Directions:

1. Boil water, and then add the turmeric and ginger. Allow it to steep for several minutes or so.

2. Filter out the herbs and combine it with honey. Blend well until the honey has dissolved, and drink it while it is hot. You can also consume it cold, but hot will work better for your back pain.

#2 Herbal Tea – Ginger and Lemongrass

So now that you understand how important ginger root can be when minimizing back soreness, please know that it can also be added to lemongrass for another effective blend for fast pain relief. Lemongrass is recognized an organic ingredient for getting rid of pain. What's even better about lemongrass is that it's easy for you to produce it in your own garden. Newly harvested lemongrass is ideal, but dehydrated lemongrass is extremely effective too if need be.

Ingredients:

1. 1 tablespoon of grated ginger

2. 2 tablespoons of lemon grass

3. 2 teaspoons of raw honey

4. 1 cup of water

Directions:

1. Bring a cup of water to a boil, and then add in your lemongrass and ginger. Remove it from the fire and allow it to steep for several minutes or so.

2. Filter out the herbs and combine it with honey. Blend well until the honey has dissolved, and drink it while it is hot.

#3 Tea - Chamomile

Quite a few men and women do not recognize that constant worry or nervousness may trigger unwanted tension and soreness in your back. An all-natural ingredient that can help alleviate this discomfort is chamomile. When added to tea, chamomile is the perfect muscle relaxant and calming agent, especially if you've had a long stressful day and need to unwind. Chamomile comes in several forms and can be purchased at just about any market or online store.

Ingredients:

1. 2 tablespoons of dried chamomile flowers

2. 1 ½ teaspoons of raw honey

3. 1 cup of water

Directions:

1. Boil your water, and then add in your chamomile flowers. Allow it to steep for several minutes or so.

2. Filter out the chamomile flowers and combine it with honey. Blend well until the honey has dissolved, and drink it while it is hot.

#4 Tea - Ginger and Spice

As you can see, there are quite a few blends that you can create to help get rid of your stubborn back pain. Adding cayenne pepper and ginger to your tea is an excellent pain fighting mixture, and it can also aid in weight loss. Combine this flavorful tea with a little bit of cinnamon to assist in soothing the aggravated muscles in your back. You can sip on this concoction all day at your job for maximum relief.

Ingredients:

1. 1 cup of water

2. ½ teaspoon of cayenne pepper powder

3. 2 tablespoons of grated ginger

4. ½ teaspoon of ground cinnamon

5. 2 teaspoons of raw honey

Directions:

1. Boil your water, and then add in your ginger and spices. Allow it to steep for several minutes or so.

2. Filter out the herbs and combine it with honey. Blend well until the honey has dissolved, and drink it while it is hot.

#5 Tea – Fennel and Cinnamon

Many people may be aware of the benefits of cinnamon when it comes to reducing soreness in your muscles, but another herb that is extremely useful also is fennel. It is excellent for pain relief and reducing stress and anxiety. When combined with cinnamon, it produces a delicious tea that can aid in eliminating long-term back aches rather fast.

Ingredients:

1. 1 teaspoon of crushed fennel seeds

2. 1 cup of water

3. 1 teaspoon of ground cinnamon

4. 1 ½ teaspoon of raw honey

Directions:

1. Boil your water, and then add in your crushed fennel seeds and cinnamon. Allow it to steep for several minutes or so.

2. Filter out the fennel seeds and combine it with honey. Blend well until the honey has dissolved, and drink it while it is hot.

#6 Tea - White Willow Bark

White willow bark is another natural anti-inflammatory that has been around for ages that you can use to minimize back soreness. If you add some honey to this blend, then you can be sure to experience some instant relief from your discomfort. But we must warn you that if you have sensitivity to aspirin, then it is not advised that you take white willow bark.

Ingredients:

1. 2 teaspoons of white willow bark

2. 1 cup of water

3. 1 teaspoon of raw honey

Directions:

1. Boil your water, and then add in your white willow bark. Allow it to steep for approximately fifteen minutes.

2. Filter out the white willow bark and combine it with honey. Blend well until the honey has dissolved, and drink it while it is hot.

#7 Tea - Lemongrass and Peppermint

A little earlier in the chapter we discussed how lemongrass can work wonders for those suffering from back problems. But another natural herb with amazing soothing properties is peppermint. The active ingredient in peppermint is menthol which produces a cooling feeling which is perfect for inflamed muscles. If you are a fan of peppermint, then this tea may become one of your favorites when you just want to relax.

Ingredients:

1. 2 tablespoons of dried peppermint leaves

2. 1 tablespoon of fresh lemongrass

3. 1 teaspoon of raw honey

4. 1 cup of water

Directions:

1. Boil your water, and then add in your peppermint and lemongrass leaves.

2. Allow it to steep for several minutes or so, and then filter out the leaves.

3. Blend well until the honey has dissolved, and drink it while it is hot.

Chapter 3

Balms That Provide Quick Relief

When flare-ups in your back occur, fast relief can never be close enough. Here are some natural home-made balm remedies that you can create and rub right in to those trouble spots. Often a person can't wait to put together a tea to drink and instead needs a faster solution. Sometimes pills and other medication may take too long to start working too. This is one of the many benefits of using balms because you can create them ahead of time, they are portable, and you can save them for quite a while for long-term usage.

#1 Balm - Cayenne Warming Balm

When seeking out the ingredients to create an effective balm for back pain, we have found that cayenne really works well. This pepper is recognized as a good healer whether you use it inside the body or on the outside. For this reason, you can use it inside a balm in addition to a tea, but you'll discover that when applied straight to your back, it'll work faster and much more effectively. The warmth will assist you to relax parts of your muscles rapidly, which could provide a fast solution to the soreness in your back. Keep in mind that this balm may not be for everyone, so make sure to test it in a small area before rubbing it all over. Make sure to wash both hands after using and make sure not to get it in your face as it could cause a burning sensation in your eyes or nose.

Ingredients:

1. ½ cup of extra virgin olive oil

2. ½ ounce of grated beeswax

3. 2 teaspoons of cayenne powder

Directions:

1. Using a double boiler, mix together the olive oil and beeswax. Stir it together over a low fire so that it mixes together. Make sure to keep stirring so it does not start to burn.

2. Sprinkle in your cayenne powder equally throughout the beeswax/olive oil mixture and stir.

3. Remove from the fire and pour into your desired containers to let cool. A tin can or glass jar that you can seal tightly is ideal. Rub into troubled sore areas on your back.

#2 Balm – Cooling Balm

As an alternative to the cayenne balm, this cooling balm can be used for back pain if you decide you do not like the heat from the cayenne. It's amazing and refreshing, and it'll assist with even severe discomfort. Make certain to use it if you feel the beginning of some discomfort coming on to for its maximum benefit. The natural healing properties of Eucalyptus oil will assist you in alleviating stiffness, in addition to peppermint and camphor oils.

Ingredients:

1. ½ cup of coconut oil

2. 2 teaspoons of grated beeswax

3. 5-6 drops of Camphor oil

4. 5-6 drops of Peppermint Essential oil

5. 5 Drops of Eucalyptus Essential oil

Directions:

1. Using a double boiler, mix together the coconut oil and beeswax. Stir it together over a low fire so that it mixes together. Make sure to keep stirring so it does not start to burn.

2. Remove from the fire and add in your Camphor, Peppermint, and Eucalyptus oils. Pour into your desired containers to let cool. A tin can or glass jar that you can seal tightly is ideal. Rub into troubled sore areas on your back.

#3 Balm - Comfrey Cooling Balm

Comfrey leaves are another all natural ingredient that can aid in easing your back pains rather swiftly. It is useful for back discomfort, bruises, sprains, as well as joint disease. It works on problem spots all over, so when you mix this into a balm, it will provide instant relief to your achy back A good idea is to add peppermint to your balm as a cooling agent which will provide an additional long-lasting effect to minimize your soreness.

Ingredients:

1. 10 drops of Peppermint Essential oil

2. ½ cup of Coconut oil

3. 2 teaspoons of grated Beeswax

4. ¼ cup of dried Comfrey Leaves

Directions:

1. Mix your comfrey leaves and coconut oil together in a medium pot over a low fire for about an hour. To avoid burning, stir on occasion and then filter out the leaves.

2. Using a double boiler, mix together the beeswax and infused oil. Stir together over a low fire and then blend in the peppermint essential oil.

3. Remove from the flame and pour into your desired containers to let cool. A tin can or glass jar that you can seal tightly is ideal. Rub into troubled sore areas on your back.

#4 Balm- Blended Arnica Balm

The power of Arnica flowers also recognized as a good pain relief remedy for back soreness. This natural flower contains properties that are very effective for pain, especially when you combine it with lavender as a calming agent. Adding peppermint also makes for a pleasant blend that will calm down any flared-up muscles in the back. Mix these ingredients together and see for yourself how much better you will feel once you rub them in to your troubled spots

Ingredients:

1. ¼ teaspoon of lavender essential oil

2. ¼ teaspoon of peppermint essential oil

3. ½ cup of beeswax granules

4. 6 ounces of dried arnica flowers

5. 2 cups of coconut oil

Directions:

1. Pour coconut oil into a large pot for an hour over a low flame. Mix in the arnica flowers and stir frequently to avoid any burning. After an hour, filter out the remaining flowers leaving behind the infused coconut oil.
2. Using a double boiler, mix together the beeswax and infused oil. Stir together over a low fire and then blend in the peppermint and lavender essential oils.

3. Remove from the flame and pour into your desired containers to let cool. A tin can or glass jar that you can seal tightly is ideal. Rub into troubled sore areas on your back

#5 Balm - Plantain Balm

A lot of folks think that plantain is a weed, but it is also a very useful ingredient for any discomfort alleviating balm. When applied topically it is proven to reduce inflammation. Plantain is also ideal for bruises and skin breakouts. Adding some peppermint oil can also add a calming benefit, along with clove oil which can be used as a numbing ingredient, which supports in expediting pain relief.

Ingredients:

1. 2 teaspoons grated beeswax

2. ½ cup of coconut oil

3. 10 drops of peppermint essential oil

4. 5 drops clove essential oil

5. ¼ cup of plantain leaves

6. 1 teaspoon of red pepper cayenne powder

Directions:

1. Pour coconut oil into a large pot and mix in the red pepper cayenne and simmer over a low flame for about 2.5 hours stirring frequently to avoid any burning.

2. Using a double boiler, mix together the beeswax and infused oil. Stir together over a low fire and then blend in the essential oils.

3. Remove from the flame and pour into your desired containers to let cool. A tin can or glass jar that you can seal tightly is ideal. Rub into troubled sore areas on your back

Salve #6 Soothing Pain Relief

Oils made from lavender are recognized for its ability to ease soreness in the muscle groups, and roman chamomile has similar properties too. It's great for relaxation and reducing inflamed muscles as well as the feelings of worry and anxiousness. Feel free to apply this mixture liberally to your strained areas.

Ingredients:

1. ½ cup of coconut oil

2. 10 drops of peppermint essential oil

3. 2 teaspoons of grated beeswax

4. 10 drops of roman chamomile essential oil

5. 15 drops of lavender essential oil

Directions:

1. Using a double boiler, mix together the beeswax and coconut oil. Stir together over a low fire until melted together.

2. Pour in your essential oils until they are thoroughly mixed. Remove from the flame and pour into your desired containers to let cool. A tin can or glass jar that you can seal tightly is ideal. Rub into troubled sore areas on your back

The Powers of Body Butter

If you are struggling with back discomfort, you sometimes simply want an exciting-natural lotion that you could apply a bit more frequently, and in most cases having a better scent. That's what these natural body butter recipes are suitable for. You can apply them to your entire back, and they are useful for other muscles that are in need of discomfort relief too. Each is intended to be used like a lotion, and contains a significantly thinner consistency than balms. However, they're frequently considered less potent, and cannot be utilized for acute back ache relief.

#1 Lavender Body Butter

Lavender body butter is simple to create, and it also has a great scent. Lavender contains properties that reduce panic, anxiousness, and stress. Chronic back discomfort is generally brought on by the tightening of muscles due to exterior reasons that contribute to stress. The properties in lavender body butter will help you take it easy to eliminate your back discomfort organically.

Ingredients:

1. ½ Cup Shea Butter

2. ½ Cup Mango Butter

3. ½ Cup Coconut Oil

4. 1 Cup Lavender Flowers, Dried

Directions:

1. With the use of a blender, blend your lavender flowers on high until they are finer.

2. Add your coconut oil in a large pot over low heat, and add in your lavender flowers, making sure they are mixed in well. Let steep over low heat for 3.5 hours, and then filter out the flowers. Keep in mind that you must stir frequently if you don't want it to burn.

3. Using a double boiler, combine all of the butters and oils together. Keep in mind that you must stir constantly over low heat if you don't want your shea butter to become gritty.

4. Allow it to cool in the refrigerator for a bit, and then remove it and whip it. Put the butter into prepared airtight containers. Apply it to sore areas as needed.

#2 Body Butter - Whipped Magnesium and Chamomile

For those who have enough magnesium, you're less inclined to experience continuous back problems, also it can aid in soothing any discomfort during flare-ups. Roman lavender flowers may also help to alleviate soreness due to its anti-inflammatory properties. You'll discover that once you infuse your oil, this mild and soft body butter has an incredible scent and it is simple to use. You are able to put it on like any other cream as often as you would like daily.

Ingredients:

1. 1 Cup Shea Butter

2. ¼ Cup Coconut Oil

3. ¼ Cup Magnesium

4. ½ Cup Chamomile Flowers, Dried

Directions:

1. Add your coconut oil to a large pot, infusing your chamomile flowers in it by simmering on low heat for 2.5 hours while mixing regularly.

2. Filter out the chamomile flowers, and add all ingredients together in a double boiler, allow it to melt over low flame while mixing to combine.

3. Allow it to cool in the refrigerator for a bit, and then remove it and whip it until it resembles butter. Put the butter into prepared airtight containers. Apply it to sore areas as needed.

.

#3 Body Butter - Peppermint and Lavender

It is already known that lavender will assist with your back discomfort, but if you add in peppermint leaves to your body butter, it makes for a powerful concoction. It'll give a cooling experience that will minimize both swelling and stiffness. Obviously, you will be reducing your tension levels simultaneously. Infuse the coconut oil for an extended amount of time if you prefer a more powerful result.

Ingredients:

1. ½ Cup Lavender Flowers, Fresh

2. ¼ Cup Peppermint Leaves, Fresh

3. ½ Cup Coconut Oil

4. 1 Cup Shea Butter

Directions:

1. In a large pot, allow your lavender and peppermint to infuse into your coconut oil by heating it on a low heat for 3.5 hours. Be certain to mix frequently to make sure nothing sticks, and then filter out the herbs, allowing the infused oil to remain.

2. Mix the infused oil and the shea butter together in a double boiler over a low flame until it melts and combines.

3. Pour it into a large bowl, whip it one time and it put it in the refrigerator to cool down.

4. When it has cooled down, remove it and whip until it is light and fluffy. Scoop it into airtight containers for use.

#4 Body Butter - Thyme and Ginger

If you don't mind the scent of a body butter that's not as fragrant, then this Thyme and Ginger combination might be just the thing to get rid of that stubborn kink in your back. It may not be as potent as some of the other body butters mentioned, but it still has the necessary properties to help alleviate chronic back pain.

Ingredients:

1. ½ Cup Thyme, Fresh

2. 4 Tablespoons Ginger, Grated

3. ½ Cup Coconut Oil

4. ½ Cup Shea Butter

5. ½ Cup Cocoa Butter

Directions:

1. Add your coconut oil to a large pot, infusing your ginger and thyme in it by simmering on low heat for 4.5 hours while mixing regularly.

2. Filter out all of the herbs, keeping the infused oil. Using a double boiler, combine the shea and cocoa butters with the infused oil.

3. Allow it to cool in the refrigerator for a bit, and then remove it and whip it. Put the butter into prepared airtight containers. Apply it to sore areas as needed.

#5 Body Butter - Lavender and Sandalwood

Similar to some of the other blends we have mentioned, anything that contains lavender will have a calming quality to it. This pleasant smelling body butter is another stress relieving combination that you can create to work into your troubled back. Sandalwood essential oil is the key component to help get rid of anxiety and stress. Create this body butter and notice the improvements you will feel to your back after you use it.

Ingredients:

1. ½ Cup Lavender Flowers

2. 20 Drops Sandalwood Essential Oil

3. ½ Cup Coconut Oil

4. 1 Cup Shea Butter

Directions:

1. Add your coconut oil and lavender flowers to a large pot and simmer on a low heat for 3.5 hours while mixing regularly.

4. Filter out all of the herbs, keeping the infused oil. Using a double boiler, combine the shea and cocoa butters with the infused oil.

2. Take off heat, pouring into a medium bowl. Add your sandalwood essential oil, making sure to combine well. Whip before placing in the fridge to cool.

5. Allow it to cool in the refrigerator for two hours, and then remove it and whip it. Put the butter into prepared airtight containers. Apply it to sore areas as needed.

Chapter 5

Amazing Bath Soaks

Some people call them bath soaks, to others they are known as bath salts, but either way they are an easy way to relieve your back discomfort. A warm bath will automatically relax parts of your muscles, however when you include herbal treatments that will help you reduce your back discomfort, it's the best! Make sure to soak for 30 or more minutes in tepid to warm water for ideal relief. If you have the time, then you can do this over the course of the day or during the night prior to going to sleep. Keep in mind that some components will loosen you up better than others, so often people choose to have a muscle relaxing bath before bed. It will help to enhance better sleep, and aid in the relief of stress throughout parts of your muscles so that you can wake up feeling renewed.

#1 Bath Soak - Tension Relaxing Salts

Dead Sea salt is ideal for the skin, and Epsom salts will assist you to relax parts of your muscles. You'll discover that the essential oils that you use are great for strain, worry, and tightness in the back. It's also going to assist with soreness, so the combination will give you a bath soak that will certainly keep the back in top shape.

Ingredients:

1. ¼ Teaspoon Roman Chamomile Essential Oil

2. 3 Tablespoons of dried Chamomile Flowers

3. ½ Teaspoon of Lavender Essential Oil

4. 4 Tablespoons of dried Lavender Buds

5. 1 Cup of Dead Sea Salt

6. 1 Cup of Epsom Salts

7. 3 Tablespoons of course Sea Salt

Directions:

1. Add all of the sea salt and essential oils into a blender on a low setting, and allow it to mix until it is smooth.

2. Mix all of the salts together in a large bowl, then pour in the dried lavender buds and chamomile flowers until it is smoothly mixed together.

3. Scoop it onto an airtight container for later use. It's recommended to use a ¼ cup to a ½ cup for each bath.

#2 Bath Soak - Ginger and Epsom Salts

A great anti-inflammatory is Ginger root, and when used as a bath salt, it can provide gentle relief for those who only have moderate back discomfort. It does not have an overbearing scent and you'll discover that it is really effective on all of the muscles when combined with the pain reducing qualities of Epsom salts. The peppermint offers a pleasant scent to this bath soak, and it'll also aid to relax parts of your back muscles and brighten up your spirits. Minimizing your anxiety levels is a terrific method to aid in reducing constant discomfort.

Ingredients:

1. 6 Tablespoons of ground Ginger

2. 10 Drops of Peppermint Essential Oil

3. 1 Cup of Epsom Salts

Directions:

1. Using a blender on low speed, mix all of the ingredients together, and then store in an airtight container until

you need it for your bath. Use a half cup with each hot bath.

#3 Bath Soak - Inflammation Reliever

If you're in search of a bath soak that may assist in alleviating any inflamed muscles you may have just a little faster, then this bath soak recipe may be perfect for you. Have you ever heard of Frankincense? No not Frankenstein. It's an essential oil that is recognized for its anti-inflammatory qualities and soreness relief. If you combine it with ginger and turmeric, it offers an effective recipe for back ache healing.

Ingredients:

1. 4 Tablespoons of ground Ginger

2. 1 Tablespoon of ground Turmeric

3. 1 Cup of Epsom Salts

4. 20 Drops of Frankincense Essential

Directions:

1. Add a teaspoon of Epsom salt and mix it with your Frankincense essential oil in a blender on a low speed. Then add in your turmeric powder and ginger.

2. Combine the blended mixture with the leftover Epsom salts. Scoop it onto an airtight container for later use. It's recommended to use a ¼ cup to a ½ cup for each bath.

#4 Bath Soak – Spasm and Stress Reducer

If you're stressed out from your day to day activities, then this could be a major reason why you are experiencing back discomfort. Improper posture while sitting, or poor lifting techniques can lead to horrible back spasms. The lavender in this back soak will help with the soreness sensation while the sandalwood oil is excellent to help keep spasms away. This bath soak is created to help prevent your muscles from feeling tight. The inclusion of Chamomile flowers adds a soothing element to the soak that assists in alleviating fear, worry, and stress. Try it out.

Ingredients:

1. 1 Cup of Epsom Salt

2. ½ Cup of Dried Lavender Flowers

3. 15 Drops of Sandalwood Essential Oil

4. ¼ Cup of dried Chamomile Flowers

Directions:

1. Combine the sandalwood essential oil with your chamomile flowers. Then add in a teaspoon of the Epsom salts and pour into a blender.

2. Stir in the leftover Epsom salts, and stir in lavender flowers. Use ¼ to a ½ cup for your bath and try to relax for at least a half an hour.

#5 Bath Soak - Nerve Pain Relief

Suffering from nerve discomfort in your back can often be difficult to relieve. Here is an effective back soak recipe that can certainly help out your aches and pains. A very useful essential oil that you can try is Juniper because it is known to target muscle spasms and nerve troubles. If you combine this oil with Sandalwood oil and thyme, it could very well be your "go to" bath soak anytime you are feeling back discomfort and need instant relief.

Ingredients:

1. 20 Drops of Juniper Essential Oil

2. 10-15 Drops of Sandalwood Essential Oil

3. 1 Cup of Epsom Salts

4. 2 Tablespoons of dried Thyme

Directions:

1. Add your thyme into a blender first to make it fine. Combine all of your ingredients together. Stir constantly to make certain that your essential oils do not clump together when mixing in the Epsom salts. We recommend you use ¼ to a ½ cup in your bath according to your pain level and how much discomfort you are experiencing at the time.

#6 Bath Soak - Earthy Pain Relief

The scent of a fresh lemon always seems to brighten up my mood, and it can work the same way for you when you are going through back discomfort. We've already discussed the magical powers of thyme when it comes to back aches, but rosemary is another natural ingredient that you can combine with it for an extra boost in pain relieving power.

Ingredients:

1. 2 Tablespoons of Lemon Zest

2. 3 Tablespoons of dried Thyme

3. ¼ Cup of dried Rosemary

4. 1 Cup of Epsom Salts

Directions:

1. In a blender, combine your Epsom salts, rosemary, lemon zest, and thyme until it's nice and fine.

2. Once it is mixed completely, keep it fresh by storing it in an airtight container. It is recommended to use ¼ to a ½ cup in your bath according to your pain level.

#7 Bath Soak - Chamomile & Peppermint

This particular bath soak formula is best for moderate discomfort. It pinpoints soreness, muscle aches, tension, and stress. The chamomile and peppermint will mask the scent of the ginger, but it will still make for quite an effective bath soak for tight back muscles.

Ingredients:

1. 20-25 Drops of Peppermint Essential Oil

2. ½ Cup of Chamomile Flowers

3. 1 Teaspoon of dried Ginger

4. 1 Cup of Epsom Salts

Directions:

1. Combine a tablespoon of your Epsom salts with your peppermint essential oil in a blender until mixed completely.

2. Blend the mixture with the rest of your Epsom salts and all other ingredients together, and keep it stored in an airtight container for freshness.

#8 Bath Soak - Lemongrass Pain Relief

This mixture can be used for more than just back problems, as it serves as a very effective pain reliever. Lemongrass is the main ingredient for helping with a sore back, but when you combine it with other essential oils such as wintergreen, you will feel its long lasting effects with this powerful bath soak.

Ingredients:

1. 10 Drops of Lemongrass Essential Oil

2. 10 Drops of Wintergreen Essential Oil

3. 4 Tablespoons of dried Lemongrass

4. 1 Cup of Epsom Salts

Directions:

1. Combine all ingredients together in a blender making sure that they are mixed well, and then store them in an airtight container for freshness. It is recommended to

use a ¼ cup to a ½ cup depending on your severity of back pain.

Chapter 6

Rub Away the Pain with Essential Oils

If you are already familiar with essential oils, then you may know how powerful and effective they can be for everyday use. Essential oils are known to be even more beneficial when you combine them into a blend. The combination of the right essential oils can target your most problematic areas of pain. Ten millimeter rollerball bottles typically work best for these essential oil blends, as it is convenient to transport and apply this way for when you may need it.

In the following essential oil recipe, we use sweet almond oil as the carrier oil. Many people also find it beneficial to use sweet almond oil mixed with coconut oil as it is also a great skin moisturizer. As soon as you start to feel soreness, it is best to apply this essential oil blend so you can start feeling instant relief.

#1 Essential Oil Blend - Calming Pain Relief

Some great essential oils that can work wonders when mixed together are lavender and valor. The scents of these essential oils are known to be powerful stress relievers and calm active emotions. The addition of peppermint essential oil will help to alleviate tight joints and muscles associated with back pain.

Ingredients:

1. 10 Drops of Valor Essential Oil

2. 10 Drops of Lavender Essential Oil

3. 5 Drops of Peppermint Essential Oil

4. Sweet Almond Oil

Directions:

1. Combine all of the oils together, and then finish it off with the blend with sweet almond oil. Shake well and apply liberally using a rollerball bottle.

#2 Essential Oil Blend - Earthy Pain Relief

Some may not enjoy the scent of this essential oil blend as much because it is rather earthy. But if it doesn't bother you much, you will find that this mixture is very effective on continuous back pain and muscle spasms. Natural ingredients such as rosemary and clary sage are noted for their relief properties when dealing with achy joints and muscles. This blend will help you to relax and it's even known to provide relief for headaches, so give it a try.

Ingredients:

1. 10 Drops of Rosemary Essential

2. 15 Drops of Thyme Essential Oil

3. 5-8 Drops of Clary Sage Essential Oil

4. Sweet Almond Oil

Directions:

1. Combine all of the oils together, and then finish it off the blend with the sweet almond oil. Shake well and apply liberally using a rollerball bottle.

#3 Essential Oil Blend - Basic Back Pain Remedy

We've discussed the benefits of lavender, ginger and peppermint when it comes to their pain relieving attributes. Combine these 3 essential oils to help ease any inflammation you may be experiencing in your back. This blend will also help to relieve tight joints along with the feelings of anxiety and stress. Go ahead and rub it in to your sore back to feel its effects.

Ingredients:

1. 20 Drops of Lavender Essential Oil

2. 8 Drops of Ginger Essential Oil

3. 10 Drops of Peppermint Essential Oil

4. Sweet Almond Oil

Directions:

1. Mix these essential oils together in a rollerball bottle, and then lastly add in the sweet almond oil. Apply generously to your troubled back areas for maximum relief.

#5 Essential Oil Blend - Numbing and Powerful Relief

Do you ever wish you could simply numb the back pain away? Well, Clove is an essential oil that can assist with that because it is known for its numbing capabilities. For this blend, we suggest that you combine it with Yarrow essential oil which helps to relieve inflamed joints and muscles. Lastly, add in some Roman Chamomile oil to complete this powerful concoction that will help alleviate back spasms and other continuous back problems.

Ingredients:

1. 10 Drops of Clove Essential Oil

2. 8 Drops of Yarrow Essential Oil

3. 10 Drops of Roman Chamomile Essential Oil

4. Sweet Almond Oil

Directions:

1. Mix these essential oils together in a rollerball bottle, and then lastly add in the sweet almond oil. Apply generously to your troubled back areas for maximum relief.

#6 Essential Oil Blend - Muscle Back Pain Remedy

Like we have mentioned before, wintergreen and sandalwood essential oils are known to help with back discomfort. Another essential oil that you can blend with the other two is White Fir. It will give your oil blend a "woodsy" scent while at the same time providing much needed relief to your chronic back pain.

Ingredients:

1. 6 Drops of Sandalwood Essential Oil

2. 10 Drops of Wintergreen Essential Oil

3. 15 Drops of White Fir Essential Oil

4. Sweet Almond Oil

Directions:

1. Mix these essential oils together in a rollerball bottle, and then lastly add in the sweet almond oil. Apply generously to your troubled back areas for maximum relief.

7 Essential Oil Blend - Nerve Pain Remedy

When you experience continuous back pain, it's not simply a tight muscle problem but more than likely a nerve issue. Juniper is a natural ingredient that will focus on those sore spots, especially when you combine it with vetiver essential oil. Feel free to add a generous amount of juniper in this combination to really aid in relieving your discomfort.

Ingredients:

1. 15 Drops of Vetiver Essential Oil

2. 15 Drops of Juniper Essential Oil

3. Sweet Almond Oil

Directions:

1. Mix these essential oils together in a rollerball bottle, and then lastly add in the sweet almond oil. Apply generously to your troubled back areas for maximum relief.

#8 Essential Oil Blend - Mood & Muscle Relief

Your mood can also have a dramatic effect on how you feel physically. Sometimes something as simple as a great song on the radio can lift up your spirit and make you forget about your pain or problems momentarily. For this oil blend, the inclusion of fresh lemon is meant to brighten your mood with its clean scent. It is then blended with marjoram essential oil and lavender which are the ingredients that will go to work on any back discomfort and stress related feelings.

Ingredients:

1. 10 Drops of Sweet Marjoram Essential Oil

2. 5 Drops of Lemon Essential Oil

3. 15 Drops of Lavender Essential Oil

4. Sweet Almond Oil

Directions:

1. Mix these essential oils together in a rollerball bottle, and then lastly add in the sweet almond oil. Apply generously to your troubled back areas for maximum relief.

#9 Essential Oil Blend - Stress & Inflammation Relief

The combinations of these 3 powerful essential oils are a perfect remedy for inflamed back muscles. As we mentioned before, Frankincense works wonders for back spasms and will help to minimize any discomfort you might be experiencing. Blend this essential oil together with sandalwood and vetiver for a calming effect to help release tension.

Ingredients:

1. 8 Drops of Sandalwood Essential Oil

2. 20 Drops of Frankincense Essential Oil

3. 4 Drops of Vetiver Essential Oil

4. Sweet Almond Oil

Directions:

1. Mix these essential oils together in a rollerball bottle, and then lastly add in the sweet almond oil. Apply generously to your troubled back areas for maximum relief.

#10 Essential Oil Blend - Lower Back Pain Relief

Many people underestimate the power of essential oils. Spruce essential oil provides great relief for muscle aches and arthritis. In this blend, we combine it with sandalwood and lemongrass essential oils which will work as a stress reliever and a muscle relaxer for your back discomfort.

Ingredients:

1. 15 Drops of Spruce Essential Oil

2. 5 Drops of Sandalwood Essential Oil

3. 10 Drops of Lemongrass Essential Oil

4. Sweet Almond Oil

Directions:

1. Mix these essential oils together in a rollerball bottle, and then lastly add in the sweet almond oil. Apply generously to your troubled back areas for maximum relief.

#11 Essential Oil Blend - Strengthened Pain Relief

Have you ever heard of Copaiba? This essential oil will provide much needed comfort as it targets inflammation in your back and reduces pain. If you enjoy a minty scent in your essential oil blend, then you will like this mix because it contains peppermint and wintergreen. This will offer a calming sensation and at the same time pinpoint your targeted trouble areas. Give this blend a try.

Ingredients:

1. 10 Drops of Peppermint Essential Oil

2. 5-8 Drops of Copaiba Essential Oil

3. 10 Drops of Wintergreen Essential Oil

4. Sweet Almond Oil

Directions:

1. Mix all essential oils together before placing in the rollerball bottle.

2. Top with sweet almond oil, and shake well before applying it to the area as needed.

Chapter 7

Effective Vitamins that help alleviate Persistent Pain

Maybe you already take vitamins as a part of your daily regiment, but there are certain vitamins that you may not be familiar with that will also help with your back problems. Even though many of these vitamins are safe to use, it's always best to check with your doctor before you start adding anything new to your system. Similar to other medicines, all-natural vitamins could potentially have unwanted side effects when mixed with other drugs. So always be sure to contact your physician before taking anything new.

Supplement #1 Vitamin D

If you have an insufficient amount of vitamin D in your system, you will definitely feel the warning signs and one of them could be consistent back pain. Taking vitamin D as a day-to-day nutritional supplement can help to alleviate your back discomfort. We suggest that you notify your doctor to help with recommending the right quantity of vitamin D you should take for your specific level of back pain.

Supplement #2 Devil's Claw

Another organic supplement that you can include into your diet regime to help relieve continuous back trouble is Devil's Claw. Harpagoside is the component in this African plant that is known for its ability to help minimize inflammation. Taking approximately fifty milligrams as part of your day to day routine will help to decrease your aches and pains in your back.

Supplement #3 Turmeric

If you open up your kitchen cupboard, I'm sure you might find some turmeric in there and that's just what you need to reduce and flare-ups in your back. Often people like to include it in their tea and drink it down. Turmeric is great for tight joints and back pain, but that saying about too much of anything isn't good for you applies here. It is also known to irritate your stomach if you use it for a long time, so be sure to use it in moderation when relieving your back symptoms.

Supplement #4 Capsaicin

If you've ever eaten hot peppers, then you may have heard that Capsaicin is the ingredient that gives peppers their spicy bite. What some people may not know is that Capsaicin is also great for minimizing back discomfort. It works by numbing the pathways that notify your brain that you may be experiencing pain. There are many over-the-counter topical forms of Capsaicin, but quite a few men and women feel that the capsule version is much more efficient when it comes to alleviating back problems.

Supplement #5 Omega-3 Fatty Acids

Adding Omega-3 fatty acids to your food plan is a good idea because it is also known to alleviate swelling which is a contributing factor to continuous back pain. Of course it is recommended to consult your doctor before you start taking this supplement to make sure it does not conflict with any prescribed drugs you may also be taking.

Supplement #6 White Willow Bark

From time to time hot tea may not do the trick and you may need a little extra boost when it comes to relieving sore muscles in your back. White willow bark is great for alleviating discomfort and has a strength similar to aspirin, but without all of the side effects. With your doctor's approval, give it a try to see if you notice any improvement in with your back issues.

Supplement #7 Bromelain

Bromelain is a natural ingredient in pineapples that has the power to decrease soreness for back pain sufferers. It is also good for those who have issues with pain in their joints and arthritis. For bromelain to be most effective, it is suggested to take this supplement with food in order for it to absorb into the body and start taking effect on your painful areas.

Supplement #8 Boswellia

People in India have been using Boswellia for generations. This native plant helps with arthritis and other ailments such as back muscles when they become inflamed. You can find this supplement in most pharmacy areas or online. To avoid a queasy stomach, be sure to take boswellia in moderation and always with food.

Remember:

Keep in mind that you should always discuss with your doctor before adding any dietary supplements to your regiment when addressing your back ache problems. Even though these are natural supplements, you never know how your body may react to them, especially if you are also taking prescription medicine. Your health care provider can discuss with you safety measures and avoiding pitfalls that are related to using multiple natural vitamins. We want you to find the right remedy to heal your back, but also want you to do it carefully.

Chapter 8

More Tips to Relieve Back Pain

You will discover that there are plenty of remedies that you could try to reduce and handle your back discomfort. Sometimes you may need to use health supplements or teas to aid you with back agony, and alternatively you'll discover there are quite a few life-style adjustments that you can develop to improve your back issues. Even long-term discomfort may be averted by means of good suggestions and improvements. These extra guidelines might help you to manage your back soreness or stop it completely. Some people may incorporate the following suggestions and way of living into any of the natural treatments that you are using currently.

Tip #1 Practicing Good Posture

Posture plays a major role in back soreness because it can also lead to more serious back spasms and episodes. Make an attempt to improve your posture whenever you notice that you are slouching or not standing straight. Make conscious attempts to improve your posture whenever you are able. It will help you to have less painful episodes while at the same time build up the muscles in your back. If you sit in a chair at work, see if you can request a more ergonomic chair to help alleviate back pain and improve posture. It that's not possible, then try using a pillow to give you the support you may need to sit correctly.

Tip #2 Regular Exercise

There are a couple of ways that exercise can help to alleviate your back discomfort. Not only will exercise make your back stronger, it will also help you to lose the weight that may be adding strain to your sore back. Starting an exercise program will drastically reduce the spasms you may be experiencing and could possibly repair your back completely. Training each day for a half an hour could have a great impact on the pain you are encountering.

Tip #3 You Could be Sleeping Wrong

Acquiring sufficient rest may help to minimize back discomfort, especially when you are experiencing continuous pain. When you experience good sleep, you are able to release tightness and tension in your back muscles. If possible, be certain to sleep on a firm bed that helps your spine rest in its natural position. You don't want to sleep in a bed that is too plush that causes your spine to sink or curve in a way that adds strain to your back. Sleeping on the wrong type of mattress could be one of the key reasons why you are experiencing back trouble. Make that change as soon as you are able and notice the natural improvements you feel to your back.

Tip #4 Meditation Works Wonders

It could appear as if meditation does not work at first glance, but truthfully it does because it helps you to calm your mind and feel focused. When your head is relaxed, the muscles in your body follow suit which also means your back will feel at ease too. Many people include meditation as a part of their morning ritual for about a half an hour every day. This practice can only help your mind and body feel better over time, especially when you combine it with other natural activities such as yoga.

Tip #5 Yoga for beginners

If you've never tried yoga before, you may want to give it a try, as many people have found it to cure their back problems. When applying yoga techniques, you improve your mobility and limberness which will assist you in preventing stress to your back during your regular routines. Yoga is also very useful in eliminating anxiety from your thoughts allowing you to feel more relaxed. Training with yoga for a half an hour to forty five minutes each day can make a substantial improvement to your back problems. It also can assist you with losing weight which can help to remove additional pressure to your achy back. It's a good idea to practice yoga when you first wake up in the morning as it sets the tone for your day allowing you to feel focused and refreshed, give it a try.

Tip #6 Stretch it Out

Occasionally the most effective component of reducing back aches is simply stretching on a frequent basis. Reach down to the floor and apply a variety of stretches to find which ones work best for you. Search on YouTube and find a ten minute stretching routine that you can incorporate into your morning schedule. If you work out day-to-day, stretching is of course a great way to begin and end your training. Some stretches may be difficult for you to perform in the beginning, but stay committed because as you become more limber, the stretches will become easier. In the end your back will thank you for it.

It Takes Time:

Keep in mind that most back issues will not fix themselves immediately, particularly if you experience from continuous back discomfort. Normally, organic treatments can deliver short-term results, but if you also use vitamins and change some of your daily habits, you'll then discover that you can have long-lasting relief. Having a conversation with your physician will help to determine the best organic cure for your back discomfort. Utilizing and experimenting with some of the remedies in this book combined with your doctor's professional advice will lead you to a stronger and more satisfied life with minimal back problems. Obviously, things will not change instantly, but remain diligent and you will gradually start to find what relief works best for you and your particular back situation.

Best of luck to you!

www.ingramcontent.com/pod-product-compliance
Lightning Source LLC
Chambersburg PA
CBHW062108280526
45788CB00003B/1395